Meditation for Beginners:
How to Calm your Mind and Reduce Stress

By Bessie Mikkel

Introduction

For many of us, we all have stressful lives. For many of us as well, we never take into account any of the various means we can use to help alleviate stress and have a much easier life. However, there are a few things that we can do which can certainly assist you in your endeavors.

One of the best ways to help improve your overall well-being and controlling your mental functions, is meditation. Meditation is a great practice, and while it is typically associated with Buddhism, it's an art and practice that is now used by many. You might have heard of some of the mind-blowing results people have gotten from this, and you might want to explore these as well.

This book will give you a comprehensive guide to meditation, including what it is, the history, some tips, and even exploring deeply the types of meditations that are out there. By the end of this book, you'll be able to understand all about meditation, allowing you to have the best results possible from your actions.

I started using meditation to help improve my life. I didn't realize that not only is it a great way to relieve stress, but also a great way to improve your life period. I wrote this book to help you with making your life much easier, allowing you to fully explore the benefits of meditation, and exactly what it could do for you.

Chapter 1: What is Meditation

The first question you might ask is what in the world is meditation? Well, there is an exact definition of this, and this chapter will go into finer detail on just what meditation is, and how it came about to be a practice that many people use today.

Essentially, meditation is a type of thought training. That might seem weird, but if you think about it, a ton of our thoughts like to come about during our daily activities. Have you ever been doing something and you get this really random, really intrusive thought that just won't go away? I'm sure that you have, and often, this can start to overwhelm our thought process, making us forget what we are doing almost. It's pretty crazy, and often, people don't realize that it actually isn't what should be happening in our daily life.

Often, many times when these thoughts come about can cause anxiety and fear in a person, and you'll end up almost forgetting what you are doing. Sometimes if it's a thought of the future, you'll be thinking about that instead of what's going on in the here and now. If it's in the past, such as maybe a regret that you might have, it can lead to you feeling sad, angry, depressed, or even jealousy. That tends to build up and boil over.

Have you ever just been irrationally angry at a person and you feel like you can't control it because your mind is focused on some anxiety-inducing problem of the past? That actually can be a result of these intrusive thoughts, and many people tend to even feel a sort of depression from this. Because of this, it prevents us from truly finding peace in the moment. If we're not focusing on the present and instead focused on the past and the future, we're letting these negative thoughts and emotions get the best of us. We shouldn't be doing that, which is why meditation is so important.

Meditation is important because it allows us to alleviate the stresses of our life and it can improve the quality of our life. It's actually not a practice that requires a ton of effort either. Instead, it's effortless and it leads to an awareness of thoughts, which means that yeah they are there, but we're not focusing on them.

Many times, people will use this to focus on the present alone, and not on the unchanging past or the future that isn't fully determined. With meditation as well, you can use different forms to really improve the quality of your life, so it's not like you're just going to use one and that's it. There are many different meditations, and they will be explored more later on.

What Meditation Isn't

Now that you know about what meditation is, let's go over what meditation isn't. Many times, people have this mindset that meditation is an effort-filled process, when in reality, it is not.

Now, meditation isn't concentration. While some might think that it is, since you're often saying a word and focusing on that word. But rather, the truth of it is, it's actually a means to not focus on these thoughts. Not all meditations are like this. Some of them are just focusing on breathing and present time. Often, the main focus is to not focus on the past, but instead just be in the present.

There is also this strange idea that meditation is loss of control. Some believe you'll lose complete control of your body, and you'll start to hear weird sounds and voices, see strange colors and pictures, or even move on your own with this sort of thing. That isn't the case. This is a loss of awareness of ourselves, and that's not what you should be focusing on. Remember, meditation is within the moment, and if you're doing that, you're not in the moment.

Now, some believe that meditation is just the breathing and posture. While these are key parts of it and help you get to where you need to go, it's not what will allow you to have the balance of your spirit. You won't be able to focus in the here and now from that alone. This is how you get started, but that isn't the end-all. We will go over posture and breathing later on, since they are important factors, but you need to have a goal with this. If your goal is to find balance and not focus on the intrusive thoughts, then that's what you go for. Your goal isn't to just sit there and look pretty, or breathe and that's it. You won't really discover the spiritual awareness that you're searching for if that's your goal, but instead it'll lead to imbalance of your spirit, which isn't what we're going for here.

Finally, it's not mental effort. You might think that it is mental effort, such as thinking "I need to not think" or the like. That isn't the case. You don't want to be held down by this, since it's actually not what meditation consists off. You want to have awareness that is thoughtless. That is what you're going for here. This needs to be effortless. It'll be natural.

Now that doesn't mean that it'll be easy. This can be quite a hard step to take, because often we're stuck in this mindset that we need to not think, and we push that forward. Instead, you just let it go, be natural, and instead you just naturally get rid of the blockages. Don't try to push the idea upon yourself that you have to do this, for it will only hurt you more in the future and lessen your progress.

That is what meditation isn't, but you've learned as well what meditation is. The next few chapters will go over some of the key points of meditation, and what you should be looking out for next.

Meditation is a spiritual practice, and it's important to know the history context behind this. This chapter will go over exactly where it came from, and how it became what it is today.

Where it Began

Now, there is speculation on what the exact date of origin of meditation is. Typically, most people assume it is around 5000-3500 BC, which is what many scholars and archeologists agreed upon due to scientific evidence. The earliest documented records of this are stemmed from the teachings of the ancient Vedas. This originated in India around this time. It was practiced by monks and holy men in the country. Throughout history, the practice was soon taken by neighboring countries, and it was soon spread around the world.

While it is now called "meditation" the word itself wasn't used until the 12th century AD. This comes from the Latin word mediatum.

The Ancient History

The records that mentioned meditation are in the Vedas. This is an ancient text that many Hindu traditions were based upon, and the Vedas actually discuss the meditative traditions. Now, while it was mentioned in these scripts, many historians can trace it way further back as well.

Now, between 600 and 500 BC, meditation started to be seen in Taoist and Buddhist India as well, and it started to spread into their practices. However, the exact origins of this practice is still debated by historians. However, the formula to salvation based on morality, concentration that contemplates, liberation, and knowledge all involve meditation as a central part of this.

Both of these religious practices do turn to meditation in order to allow the person to reach the highest level of spiritual awareness possible.

Later on, meditation was seen in other practices as well. In *The Yoga Sutras of Patanjali* it outlines the eight limbs of yoga and the theory behind it. This was compiled between the 400-100 BD era. During this time, another document was written, called *Bhagavad Gita* which talks more about the philosophy of yoga, spirituality, and also meditation and how all of these work together.

Now, meditation spread to the west and further east due to the Silk Road. It actually has some influence in western religions such as Judaism. It was even seen in Christian faith in a sense, for Plotinus in the 3rd century AD actually created meditative techniques that weren't easily integrated, but still used by many. His type of meditations were called "spiritual exercises" which involved using concentration. While some did use them, they didn't attract a following among various meditators. However, Saint Augustine did try to experiment with this on him in order to see if they achieved ecstasy.

The transmission of Buddhism actually ended up bringing meditation over to other oriental countries. There was another school that came forward as well, called Zhiyi in the 6th century, and this managed to take the teachings that were imparted and soon, it ended up creating a relationship that made more sense. It even evolved in Korean Buddhism in the 7th century.

Now in the east, a Japanese monk by the name of Dasho, discovered the practice of Zen when he visited China in the year 653 AD. Eventually, this also brought in the practice of meditation to Japan when he got back. He ended up opening the first meditation hall there. Eventually, the practice grew even more to the point that in the 8th century AD, it was seen as a common practice to meditate in the land.

Now it wasn't called meditation until about 400 years later. Again, the word originates from Latin, which means "to ponder" and a monk named Guigo II actually introduced this for the first time around that era, which changed everything.

From the Middle Ages to Modern History

Now, meditation spread to the west through Judaism and through the people of Europe meeting those in the east as well. Throughout the middle ages, meditation actually grew and became more popular with many people. This was actually a key component of prayer and Jewish meditation, which was often done by many people. Despite being heavily Christian, the process of meditation was integrated in order to help bring a heightened sense of spirituality to many people.

In Christianity, this type of meditation was often seen in a sense of saying the same phrase while maintaining a posture, which actually can be seen all the way back to the byzantine era. However, western Christian meditation actually contrasts with these other approaches since it doesn't have the repetition of the actions nor does it require posture. However, western Christian meditation was actually still used even in the 6th century, with many people reading the bible in a divine sort of manner. Many Benedictine monks used this, and many saints including Ignatius of Loyola and Teresa of Avila in the 16th century used meditation in order to help contemplate, pray, and read more in order to gain a heightened sense of spirituality.

Now, it only continued to grow and grow until about the 18th century, when ancient teachings became more popular in western cultures, and from this, the boom in meditation began.

For many during this time, the study of this was actually a topic that many philosophers and intellectuals decided to take ups, such as Schopenhauer, and even Voltaire. Voltaire himself asked for toleration towards those that practice Buddhism and did encourage this in his teachings.

There we also schools of yoga that came about because of the Hindu revivalism that happened in the 1890s. Some of these schools started to come to the west by many famous gurus. Many however were started to be promoted as secular versions of yoga traditions used by many that weren't Hindus, such as transcendentalist meditation. There are also various yoga schools that have started to come forward, and in the western world, the practice of both meditation and yoga has become extremely popular.

Now the real focal point to modern meditation practice is actually found in 1927. This is in the book called "Tibetan Book of the Dead." It was published, and it immediately got a lot of attention from westerners, and it sparked them to be interested about the practice. Now, this then spawned into the *Vipassana* movement, which is essentially insight meditation. This began in Burma during the 1950s, and this also led to further literature being published around this time, such as "The Dharma Burns" which was put out in 1958. This brought more attention to meditation as well.,

Now, it even got into medical practices as well, for in 1979 it ended up being part of a stress reduction program in the US, which constituted of people using meditative techniques to help various patients that suffered from chronic diseases, to many great results.

Now, since then it's actually become so common that about 10% of the American populace now meditates. While it is Hindu in origin, it actually plays a key role in many rituals and traditions of various other religions, but it is also used by those that don't practice religion in order to help them keep their stress levels down and even improve their overall happiness and well-being as well.

From this, you can see that meditation has a very rich and interesting history. Through this as well, you can see just how far-reaching meditation can be to help a person, and the spiritual awareness that a person can have from this as well. It's a practice that's been used for thousands of years, and it can be used by you to help you out in many different ways.

Now for many people, they are skeptical of meditation, for often they don't realize what it can do for themselves. However, exploring this concept can generate a lot of very interesting results, and while these are benefits, you might start to realize within yourself just what meditation can do. While this isn't the end-all to what meditation can help with, it certainly can lead you down the right path and allow you to fully obtain the benefits of this type of practice, and all that is associated with this.

Emotions Under Control

Now, many times, we are caught up in the emotions of the world. We might end up feeling this in our daily life, whether it be from others, or eve from ailments that might be there. Many times, the world is painted as a very dismal place. However, we don't have to always feel that way.

Many times, the reason why we feel this way is because we succumb to the societal emotions that are out there. Often, people love to paint the world as a terrible place, always destructive, and the like. However, if you don't succumb to this, you can often feel better. Depression, sadness, and the like are often emotions that can control you. Bad situations do happen, but your response can determine the fate that you will have. With our emotions, we tend to not fully place them under our thumb, and when they run wild, we might end up saying things we don't mean to say, which in turn can cause us to lose friends, relationships, and we could even hurt our future.

With meditation, we're taking the time to actually look at these emotions that we're focusing on, and from there, we can place them under our control. It can help with anyone who is prone to extreme anger in situations, where they might end up reacting in an unfavorable way. For many people, this can make a difference in their future, and meditation will allow these concentrative factors to come forward, and you can put them under your control in due time.

Physical Ailments and Meditation

Now and interesting point to consider is that sometimes, the reason why we succumb to ailments is because of our emotions and the turmoil of this. Now, not all illnesses are caused by extreme emotions. You might be around a substance that you're allergic to, and that can cause problems. But if you've ever experienced violent mood swings, hallucinations, depression, and the like, this can be traced to emotions as the root. In some cases, it can cause actual tissue damage, such as in the case of extreme stress. If you take a look at this, many diseases often have at the root disruptive emotions that we don't have under control. There are programs that can help relax you, and one of them is meditation.

If you are able to control these emotions, it can often control these physical effects. For example, let's say you have ulcers that are flaring up constantly whenever you're really angry. With meditation, you can actually relax the body, and control that disruptive thought, allowing the prevalence of those ulcers to become less and less apparent.

In Buddhist tradition, it actually is used to get rid of the source of any trouble in yourself, which then can help one overcome the thoughts that they have. Now, if you get rid of these emotions, you'll start to notice that it actually allows you to have a true illusion of yourself, seeing this there, which in turn will help you get rid of the negative emotions, which can cause physical illnesses to come about. It can also change the way you view yourself, allowing you to realize just what kind of person you are.

Reducing Stress

Another great thing that meditation can do for you, is to help eliminate stress. Stress is often caused by someone focusing too heavily on a disruptive thought, and because of this, it often will cloud the way a person views themselves. With stress, it ends up becoming the forefront of our thoughts, which in turn is extremely intrusive and not helpful whatsoever. With meditation, we'll be able to focus on ourselves, fixing up the way we think, and even changing the way we view one another. Meditation can ultimately change the future of our thought process, and if we're able to relax, we'll be able to have much less stress as well.

Controlling Negativity

We often have a load of negative thoughts about ourselves. Self-confidence can often be crushed because of the accumulation of negative thoughts. However, what if you could take those negative thoughts and make them go away, or control them enough so that they're not causing you a burden? That's the point of meditation, for if you control those thoughts, you can ultimately control the way you view yourself.

Many of us have a poor outlook on ourselves and it's because focus on what was said in the past by others, whether it be positive or negative. If you've been told that you're ugly in the past, chances are you'll focus on that sometime in the future. If you are able to harness these thoughts and control them, you'll start to realize that those thoughts are the reason why you've held yourself back, and it can be almost life-changing if you begin to realize this. That's why it's important to focus on the here and now, and not on past thoughts, for it can make or break your self-confidence in a sense, and meditation can help with this.

Stabilizes Yourself

Now, according research by Pavlov, everything is interconnected. The production of hormones is related to the body, and even how you act and react to situations. Every part of a person is related to one another, and it's why your thoughts and emotions have such huge effects. Your thoughts have power. If you think you won't make it, you won't. If you think you're going to get emotional if you hear this, then chances are, you will end up getting emotional. Emotions and thoughts are so far-reaching that they can control a person.

However, with meditation, you're calming the body down, changing your focus to your life and not letting this whole cacophony of thoughts and emotions worry you. You'll start to have a much healthier thought process too. That's why it contributes to good health, and it can even bring about a much healthier sort of body for yourself.

Changing Your Physical Characteristics

Meditation can even change your physical characteristics. Now, this can be in terms of how your blood pressure and heart rate are. For many, just sitting there and focusing on it will relax and calm the body. If you live a life that is riddled with stress, you might have high blood pressure, which leaves you open for heart disease, the number one killer in the world today. However, sitting there and calming yourself down can help you lower this, allowing you to have a longer life.

Many people don't realize how much stress they have until they sit for five minutes and meditate. It's magical, and it can change you.

This can even change your health as well. Many people tend to want to do things better for themselves because of the increased mindfulness of their body. People don't realize just how much garbage they're putting into their body, and how much they rely on substances such as alcohol and cigarettes. You'll realize just how harmful these are to your body, and how natural foods feel. You might realize this while mindfully eating one day that "hey, this isn't that bad. I feel more energy" and you might cut out processed foods entirely. Now this is obviously your decision, but it can change your overall health outlook as well.

You can even slow down aging and your immune system as well. Because of your cognition of all that is going on, you tend to realize how your body looks a bit more. There are studies that show that meditators tend to have longer telomeres, which are caps on chromosomes that indicate your biological age. It can help you if you want to look younger for longer. While actually living longer is a stretch, it can slow down your aging since there is much less stress on the body.

When it comes to your immune system, you'll realize as well that your body actually isn't getting as sick as much. Think about it, because you're harnessing these negative emotions and intrusive thoughts, you won't be susceptible to stress, and from there sickness. If you've been worried about the state of your immune system, consider relaxing a bit, for it can change you.

How Meditation Changes Self

Meditation can change the way you look at yourself. Self-awareness is something that many people don't really pay enough attention to, allowing ignorance and the like to be at the helm. But of course, what if you spent a bit more time looking at this? Well, self-awareness can allow you to realize two things: what you're doing to yourself, and what is stopping you from being happy.

Meditation allows you to recognize your anger, your depression, and your own emotions, and you can become detached from this. Your mind will feel clearer, and it will calm you down. You'll feel more comfortable in your own skin, and you'll realize just who you really are. Coming to terms with the truth about yourself and accepting it is often something that is a huge problem for many. We love to paint a picture of ourselves that we feel is right, but ultimately, it isn't. However, meditation allows you to see the reality of this, and change it to best fit you.

With that as well, you'll start to realize that you are happier. Now, there are studies that have demonstrated that there are increases of left brain side of your cortex, which is where the positive emotions are. The right side decreases, which is where the negative emotions are. This is because you're taking the time to harness this, and when you become more self-aware, you start to feel happier, and you have an overall better well-being. Happiness is really based on you, and you determine your own happiness. By using meditation to help harness the negative emotions, you can change your entire outlook on life from this alone, and in truth, that can really make a difference in the way you feel about your life, and how you go about living it.

Meditation can do so much for you, as demonstrated in this chapter. From health, to even your overall well-being, you can change this for the better using meditation. It's up to you what you do with this, and you'll begin to see from here just what it can do to change you for the better, and what it can make you feel as well.

With meditation, there are three types of out there that can actually help you. You might actually be indulging in one of these without realizing what it is. This chapter will go over the three different types, and how each of them work.

Typically, in our society we don't realize we're doing this, and typically we end up thinking we have to have a set time to meditate. The truth is, these various forms of meditating can actually be done on your own volition, and while some might use these for religious traditions, they can also be used to help you with your own daily struggles. You'll learn with each of them what they are, and why it's important to understand each of them, and a few examples of what they can be.

Concentrative

This is probably the easiest one to understand, and it's probably the one that you've done before, or at least seen. Essentially, it's a type of meditation where you concentrate on your surroundings. Your goal with this is to actually focus on the action at hand, and not letting the intrusive thoughts that might come about.

Now with concentrative meditation, this is actually a means of focusing on something that is specific. For example, let's say that you want to use a mantra. Or maybe you want to repeat a word to yourself, or even breathing, this is what it all falls under. The basic meditation techniques typically fall under this umbrella, and they're used to help you concentrate on your surroundings and not let these intrusive thoughts get the best of you.

You can even look at a candle flame if that's what you're going for here. The ultimate goal is concentration, and you just want to let the thoughts come and go, not letting your mind get hung up in them. That's what you're going for here. This can even be applied to life. For example, let's say something happens in the workplace, or you get some bad news. Often, it's a natural response to lash out, feeling angry and hurt, and you might even feel vengeful. However, if you use concentrative meditation, you want to instead take the negative incident, and let it not get the best of you. If you do, it will end up controlling you, and you might even be bent on revenge, which isn't a healthy sort of means of coping at all. Planning and plotting revenge has you focused on the past, and not on the present, which can lead to overall unhappiness.

Now instead, with concentrative meditation, if you get a bad situation that rears its ugly head, you want to instead just note that this is happening, and instead refocus your attention so that you can actually handle the bad experience and not get stuck in the dream. That's why the focusing on your breathing is used, or the candle, or the chant. If you do focus on the drama, you won't be able to achieve true happiness, but instead you'll wallow in your grief.

This is a type of practice used by many yogis and monks. Now, not everyone is perfect, but remember, if you can control your emotions, even just a little bit, think of how you might respond to situations better, how different everything might be for you, and your overall happiness. It can make a huge difference, and it can certainly make you feel fuller of life as well.

With this as well, you can even include music as well if it is hard for you to keep your thoughts to yourself. It's a good way to focus, and you'll be able to really feel the results of your actions as well as you go along.

Meditative Movement

For many people, it's often hard for them to just sit and be there. They don't want to just sit around and meditate, even if it is for a couple of hours. However, movement meditation is actually a great means to help overcome this. Now, the cool thing about this, is that you don't have to have any huge instructions, other than you need to move. However, it's important that you do have a mindfulness associated with this, where you do focus a little bit on what movements you are doing.

Now with movement, you can do whatever you want, such as shaking your body, dancing, or whatever you like. You should do this in a space with nobody else around, since it can be a bit of a self-conscious point, since some might find it a bit strange. You should do this for about five minutes, and if you feel like you need to continue do so. Often, some people like to do this to help themselves focus on their body and the movements of this.

When you are done, go sit still for a few minutes. You can stand as well if you really feel it, but be comfortable. You should pay attention to what your breathing is doing. You might end up being surprised at what might come up, such as emotions that might come about. This can also happen especially with shaking and dancing if you do it for a bit. Many times, we have repressed emotions that can typically not show up until you really dive into them. This isn't bad.

Now if you do become emotional during this, it's actually healthy for you. However, if it becomes more powerful, you might need to couple this with more breathing. If it is a lot, you might have other discomfort issues that you might need to work on yourself. But getting emotional during this type of movement is often a normal thing, and not something to worry about. This is a great way to help you get unstuck from your thoughts, or make you feel like you're somewhere else as well.

For some people, you can even couple this type of movement with martial arts. If you do yoga, martial arts, or even tai chi, you can do this with meditation movements. It can even make you feel like you're a new person because of it. If you do choose to mix in this ancient discipline with even some meditative movements, you'll start to notice that your body is much freer. You can do this with various postures and detailed movements, and it can even demonstrate a sort of harmony between both of these realms, giving you a chance to really improve on this.

If you've done martial arts or tai chi before, try to focus on your movements and just work on these techniques, paying attention to how your body is and the meditative effects of it. It might be the right thing for you, and there are also other people out there that can help you with this, such as those that run classes in tai chi and martial arts, which is an option as well.

Expressive Meditation

This is the last category of meditation that you'll learn about in this chapter. Essentially, this is a great means for those that are creative to get into meditation. This involves creating a sort of place to let your creations run wild. For many people, this is forcing more on right hemisphere activities, which is where much of the creativity resides.

For many people, movements and breathing are great, but sometimes people feel a bit stumped on creativity. We've all been there before where we feel like we're doing something, but then our creativity gets smothered because of societal expectations. If you feel like your thoughts are all over the place, or maybe you just feel stumped on creativity, you might want to consider exploring this. There are many ways to get into it, such as using a journal, drawing, working with sand, stone, or even sticks, and using your hands to create what you want. In our lives, we've been told time and time again what we can't create, and how people frown upon art and such. We might be artists ourselves, but we haven't been able to channel that energy due to the lack of concentration to the task. However, expressive meditation allows you to focus on that, using music and other means to help you keep your concentration there.

If you want to journal, you can always do that. You just spend some time alone, holding the journal out, and start to just write down how you feel about anything. This doesn't have to be a set topic, but instead write what you feel comes up. For some, it can be about the events that happened, such as maybe emotions tied to an event, or other times, it's mostly the freedom to express emotion. Often, we hold ourselves back from truly expressing ourselves, and it's seen in many sorts of ways. Often, we don't let ourselves actually come forward and feel what we want to feel, so this is a great way to push that forward.

You can, if you need structure, talk about the thoughts and feelings that you have for that day, or even writing about a particular topic. If you have for example, some sort of chronic illness, sometimes getting the feelings associated with that out of your mind on the daily can help with making that illness less of a problem. It's mind-blowing what this can do for you, and it makes everything so much better as well.

If you are the type of person that often has the notion to always stop and think about what you need to say, or holds yourself back from truly saying what they want to feel because of their mind, then it's important to try this. Many times we want to say what we want to say, but often, because of societal expectations, or maybe your grammar or the subject matter can cause us to not want to really push this forward. However, if you want to really get a stronger insight on the situation, it will allow you to feel a bit more relaxed, and less stressed out about everything at hand.

Now, you have seen here the three types of meditation. Remember, this actually can all be used at the same time if you truly feel like you need to, or you might choose one and not the other two. Whatever it might be, do pick one that best fits your situation, and begin to use this daily. You'll feel the difference in the results right away if you do this, allowing you to have a freer life that is definitely much more liberating for you.

Chapter 5: Meditation Tips for Beginners

Now, when you're beginning, there are often a few tips that people push onto those that begin to meditate that they believe are the truth and only the truth. Now, this isn't the case, and before we begin talking about the types of meditation, we'll start with discussing some of the important tips to keep in mind that you should know about when you start.

The first, is that you can do this anywhere. That's right, you've probably had the idea that you need to do it in some weird position that is incredibly uncomfortable. Well guess what, you can actually do this anywhere, any time of the day, and in various positions and forms. We'll go over a few of the great ones to start with, but you'll be able to really get the most benefits if you realize that you don't need to be held to the idea that you must close your eyes and say "omm" when you do this. That's not true, and in fact, it's much simpler than that.

Another common misconception that people have is they must meditate with their eyes closed. That actually is a huge misconception, and in fact, it's harder if you start with your eyes closed. While it is acceptable for you to have your eyes closed when you sit and meditate, often if you're just starting out, you'll end up dozing off if you're not careful. That's a common problem that many people start with, so it's actually much better for you to have your eyes kind of open, since it'll help with keeping alertness high without falling asleep. There are some meditations that work with the eyes partly open as well, and some don't even close them, so keep that in mind.

Now, when you begin, you might think that you should do one of those complex and really thought-out meditations, but guess what, you might actually end up getting yourself totally unfocused, and you won't be as happy with the results as say if you started a bit simpler. Walking meditations, mindfulness meditations, and the like are definitely much harder on the spectrum of meditation than simple breathing ones. It's important you start off easy, such as using mindful breathing. If you do this, even if it's for a few minutes, you'll see the results right away. Even something as simple such as mindful breathing, which is basically sitting down and meditation while you're mindful of your breath for a minute or two will prove to have much more spectacular results that you might think. Start with what works for you.

Now, if you start to feel an energy in your body as you meditate that makes you feel antsy, that's actually a common symptom of it working. If you're restless as well, it often can hinder your progress. If that's the case, you shouldn't force this. You can then walk and meditate, such as walking in a slow manner with mindfulness. We'll go over walking meditation more later.

Often, people think they should just sit there and get through it. However, sometimes that doesn't go away, and you might feel that energy as a sign of a new mindfulness. Getting rid of it will allow you to sit much better. In the beginning, you should sit for as long as you can, and that restlessness should be pushed through, but if you've been consistently doing this and you still find yourself a bit restless, do take the time to do some walking meditation and then sit after. This can be a sign of an increased level of awareness, which isn't a bad thing either, and sometimes that awareness energy needs to be dealt with accordingly.

You should also figure out what works for you. This means that if you've started with the beginner activities and you've done it for a bit, try other types of meditation. For example, if you have done some breathing ones, you might start to do driving, eating, and walking meditation. With this, it's actually limitless, and there are a few other techniques that will be explored later on, but the best thing to do is to find out what works best, and start to structure the type of meditation that you do based on this. You should choose what works for you.

If you're a fan of sitting and meditation, you can still do that, but don't do it for half of a day, but instead switch it up and do some other meditations that are out there that works for you. If you feel like you need a bit of a push, this is a great way to get started with it, so do consider it.

Now, people think that meditation will come to you right away. That isn't always the case. Sitting down and just relaxing, not focusing on anything, can be quite hard. Our minds are always focused on something, and typically they like to run at a speed where it's as if they are a computer and have forty tabs open. Many times it's very difficult for someone to get breathing meditation down, but that's actually natural. For some, it might be a bit easier to be mindful, but not for others. You shouldn't get discouraged or think that you'll never get it if you don't do so right away. This is challenging, but if you give up, you're only evading the benefits that you could get on this.

Now when it comes to focus, you shouldn't have a hard focus. For many of us, we try to focus on something so hard that it actually becomes tiresome. If you're being mindful, you should have a focus that is constant, but not super hard, on the obvious that you're using. You should do this with anything that comes into your awareness. For example, maybe you hear the phone ringing while you're doing a breathing meditation, or you see a squirrel while doing a walking one. Don't make that the hard focus, because it'll hurt your eyes and hurt your brain. Instead, just focus on it for a second and let it go away. You should instead acknowledge it, but then go back to your meditations. The same with breathing. Know that it's there, but don't put emphasis on this.

When you are doing this, often we begin to obsess over whether or not we're doing it correctly. However, that isn't the way to do it. It does take time to master, but instead of thinking whether you're doing it right or not obsessively, you should get the instructions that you have and just simply follow them. Do a little bit every single day.

As long as you do this and just do that, you don't need to obsess over whether you're doing this right or wrong. That's a big problem with many who begin. They tend to love to obsess over the right or wrong ways. We're a society that obsesses over doing everything right, and while that is often a good thing in some cases, it's not what you should be focusing on when you're meditating. You should just do what it says and not worry about anything else.

For many people, there is also the worry about their hands. You've probably seen all those fancy little pictures where people are doing something with their hands. It's an interesting position, and it's called a mudra. It's a sign that means that it's an important part of a meditation or a spiritual tradition. Now, these can help the practice when you're sitting, and if you want to use them, go for it, but they aren't required. Just remember that if it's extremely distractive, it's probably better to not do it.

Finally, you should definitely be alert to a degree while you do this. This is a literal meaning to waking up. When you first start meditation, you'll want to doze off. Some people tend to do that a lot with sitting meditation. If you're prone to this, you'll want to change your routine up to accommodate this factor. You can also drink something with caffeine, or do it at a different time to help you really get the most out of this. You will want to figure out what is right for you. If you're a person who is more aware during the morning, meditate in the morning, and you should do it when you have full energy and when you're not feeling sleepy anymore. This is how you'll get the most out of your meditations, allowing you to be even more successful.

These tips will help anyone with getting started. It's not hard to begin, but it often does take a bit of a push. If you give yourself the right push, you'll be able to get the results from this immediately. Take the time to fully educate yourself on this, and follow these tips, for they will make meditation all the more easier.

Now, before you begin, you should make sure that you are prepared to meditate. Preparing for meditation can make a difference in your ability to meditate, and this chapter will go over what you can do in order to fully attain the best benefits that you can, and why posture matters when you're trying to have the best meditation experience that you can have.

Posture Matters

To begin, you need to have a room that isn't full of drafts that could distract you, isn't cluttered, and in general isn't too loud or anything. You should do this in a place that is free from distractions. If you have a phone, keep it over to the side, and make sure that you do it on a regular sort of schedule. If you get cold, you should bring a blanket as well, and if it's warm outside, adjust the A/C accordingly and have a blanket on hand.

Now, the key component here is that you do this at your own comfort level. Make sure that this is a schedule that you're able to do, and make sure to keep it. You should make sure you sit down in a manner so that you're not in pain or feeling discomfort, and you should find the right posture that you can hold for a period of time. You should try to be straight, but if you can't fully keep straight for whatever reason, make sure that you're relaxed. Try not to control, nor try to expect anything. Just be there.

When you do this, wear clothing that is loose and comfortable, and you should try to wear as little as you can. If you wear a belt or anything distracting such as a bra, do try to loosen it as you can. If you wear a watch or some jewelry, take it off. If you tend to wear perfume, don't do so during that time, since it is actually distracting. You don't need to have adornments during meditation, so try to avoid it.

Legs

If you're worried about your legs, just try to be as comfortable as possible. Some people try to do the full-lotus, but if you can't due to your lack of flexibility, don't get all hung up on it. However, below are the steps to get into the full lotus position effectively.

- Sit on the floor or on a cushion if you need it with your right leg in front and then pull it close to where your groin is.
- Take the left leg and put it over it, with the left foot resting with the sole of your foot upwards, on your right thigh and close to where your groin is.
- Then, take your right foot, with the sole up, and then put it onto the left thigh, trying to bring it as close to the groin area as you possibly can.

Now this is something that if you don't have the flexibility for it, it can be quite hard. You however want to stay in this position for some time if you want to focus more on how you sit. However, you should do this for a short period of time.

You might end up getting used to this, which is totally fine, and if you so desire, you can sit like this for the duration of your meditation. You don't even have to do this if you don't want to, but some find it helps with the quietness, stability, and the tranquility of sitting, so they might encourage it.

You can do the half-lotus position, however, it doesn't give you a firm base, since one knee is weighed down instead of two legs. But, for flexibility reasons, some might not be able to do this. However, one way to help compensate for this to help you achieve better flexibility, is to switch the position of your legs as you sit down, and with every single sitting, which at the onset might be no more than a couple of minutes.

If this is too hard for you to do immediately, you should set some time aside to stretch out your muscles in the leg area, groin area, and the hips, however you should make sure that you do take you time with this and don't pull a muscle, since that can take a long time to recover. What you should do is try the half-lotus with each leg as much as you can, and do it in a gradual and steady manner. By doing this, you'll start to become much more longing, patient and you'll begin to understand yours and you'll feel more relaxed. You however shouldn't force yourself into a position if it brings you pain, since there are misalignments and twists that can happen, and those are very uncomfortable. Do what is right for you, and you'll feel much better.

If you need help with loosening the muscles that keep your legs from being on each side so that they can rest on the floor, is to get a meditation seat. These are available at the store, and you can sit on the very edge of it with the knees about the width of the shoulders apart and your knees over your ankles. You can then take one leg and put the ankle on the side of the other, and then you can let the knee move out as far as it can go with it being supported by your hand, and then lift and lower it again. Each time you do it, picture the leg relaxing more, and then set it down again and let it go each time, feeling what you might need to do to have this happen. Keep your hips at level the entire time and that your legs can sink lower and lower. Do be mindful the entire time of everything that is going on when you do this. If you can't manage to sit in these, you can sit in the free position.

If you feel pain start to come about, don't do it. If you see this, rather than complaining about it and wishing you were somewhere else, will help you a lot more. Don't try to brave it, but instead just stay with it and observe it. You will soon see how you can make the effort much easier, and you might even observe what is going wrong, allowing you to change the outlook of the situation.

With anything that happens here, you should observe and allow this to happen. Don't try to avoid it or not face it, but instead just take it in. Even if you want to leave, you should be mindful of what's going on, since you're the only one in touch with yourself, and exploring this makes all the difference.

With anything that you do in this, you should always look at the response that you're giving and also send love and kindness to yourself. You might end up feeling emotional, find this silly, or even embarrassing, but if you do practice this type of loving kindness, you'll have a simple and profound means of reaching to the deepest part of yourself and addressing this. You should have an insightful meaning to this, which we'll go into further detail later on.

If you do end up finding the pain too distractive, you should consider it, rather than have it in a kindness manner. You should see that it is there. If you need to stretch out your legs mindfully, do so, and then rest and return to this. Your goal is to sit correctly and not get involved in sitting correctly, since it'll allow you to achieve much more, and you'll start to notice that not only will it become quiet, but your breathing will be much subtler and the muscles much more relaxed, and it will allow you to have a natural meditation.

Chest, buttocks, and abdomen

These are the last areas to focus on. You should take the time to raise your chest, moving it forward, and sit so that the hollow of your chest, which is right near where your sternum is, allows your diaphragm to function without anything wrong. If you're new to meditation, you might find discomfort and obstruction sitting like this, and that's because your heart den isn't low enough. If this does occur, focus on the abdomen and don't put any effort. Just acknowledge that it is there, and soon, you'll feel much better as well.

With your butt, you should have it protruding a little bit, with your back comfortable and erect. You should be working to sit relaxed and composed, allowing it to settle into your lower abdomen, which is especially calming.

Now, with your hands, if you're wondering what to do with them, initially, don't worry so much about it. However, if you so desire, you can sit with the palms turned up, and with the back of your hand resting on the palm of where your left us, and the back of the left can sit at the lower part of your abdomen.

This might feel a bit strange, but you should do what you feel is natural and uncomfortable. If you don't feel like this is how you want to sit, then don't do it. It's up to you whether you want to or not.

The way you sit can determine how your meditation sessions go, and while comfort is at the forefront, there are ways to help promote this and make it even better for you. This chapter allowed you to explore this, allowing you to have a much better sort of mindset when it comes to meditation, allowing you to have much more success as well.

Breathing is the next part of this, and it's important to realize that breathing is an integral part of this, since it allowed you to focus. This chapter will highlight various breathing techniques to keep in mind, and why you must do so.

Natural Breathing and Why It's Important

The key breathing that you should be doing when you're meditating is natural breathing. This is essentially when you relax as you inhale and then contract as you exhale. Your lungs will expand as you inhale and contract as well when you exhale. This is natural since the diaphragm will move upwards in the chest, and the abdomen contracts because of it. This will help in evacuating the lungs of anything that isn't supposed to be there, but it also will get the blood flowing to various parts of the body that need it, since you're compressing the viscera.

Right Breathing

Now, there is another method of breathing if you want to try something different, and it requires a bit more work, but it can help clear the mind better, and it actually can bring more air to the body as well. This is called right breathing. Essentially, the abdomen contracts when you inhale and relaxes as you exhale. This type of breathing is old, and it's been around in ancient China for many years. It is used to help improve the physical and mental capabilities of someone.

Now, this is definitely something you need to consider for yourself. For many of us, choose the one that best fits you. If you get caught up in your breathing being a certain way, you'll end up getting obsessive over it, which in turn will reduce the effects of this and make them slightly less effective.

Why practice Breathing

You might want to consider practicing this, and this is where you begin to learn something new about yourself. When you are relaxed, it becomes much more evident that your breathing is going on, and you know that it's going on. You can also breathe in a certain way intentionally, but the need to do so is really based on the circumstances outside that require this intention, so you're not really needing a bunch of choice in the matter. You should breathe how you believe it should be naturally done. Remember, with meditation, you do this in the absence of thought, and yet we think as well that without thought there would be no meditation. In a sense, you're trying to think, but not to think, and that creates an interesting conundrum, since these are two separate things rather than what is apparent.

If you're paying attention to your breathing, you're not necessarily calm, so you should relax so that you can be calm. Meditation without thinking and your breathing itself are both kind of in the same sort of vein, since you want to not think about this. In this sort of thing, you don't want to have control. You want to bring about a state of relation in almost a circuitous manner, and in a sense by doing so you're also using your will. There is also a rule that holds true, whether you're doing one type of breathing or another. You should in practice always sit erect breathing through your nose. You can exhale through your mouth, but again, that's putting more thought onto the body, so it's not encouraged.

You might notice as you practice this that your breathing is shallow and rapid. However, as you relax, you might start to notice that you're not accepting or rejecting whatever shows up, and your breathing will slow down and deepen at one point. You might notice that the cycle goes on for a long time, almost once every minute. You might consider this to be a sort of standard in a sense, making sure that you're not forced or uncomfortable, but instead you do this naturally without any concern on your part.

However, you might notice that as you sit down and do this, your breathing is much finer. If you are going to participate in meditation, you should consider devoting at least a few minutes every single morning to this type of breathing practice. By doing this, you'll start to notice the finalities of your own breathing, and you can practice this multiple times during the day, whenever you think about it. This can also help if you start to feel anxiety about something as well, for it can help alleviate the tensions there.

You might notice that as your breath slows and becomes much subtler, the mind will stabilize and calm down. Remember, as the mind goes, so does the breath in a sense. In a sense, your breathing goes about in four stages, and it's important to realize that these four stages are there for a reason.

Four Breathing Stages

These four stages are important to realize, for they can help you master the art of breathing. Breathing in it of itself is something that you should realize, and by doing so, you'll be able to notice how the mental changes come about as a result too.

- Windy breath: this is the first stage, and you might notice this immediately. This is when you sit and hear almost a windy sound when you're breathing. That is the natural sound of your breath.
- Gasping breath: this is stage two, which is where you won't make sounds when you breathe but you have the feeling that you're not truly taking in enough.

- Air breath: this is the third stage and the third type, where the breath is silent and even without any obstruction to this, however you're not totally calm there. It feels clear as the air, and often, you'll notice that while you've achieved this stage, there are still signs of unrest there.

- Silent breath: this is the final stage of this, where you will notice that you don't feel like you're breathing at all in a sense. There isn't a roughness of softness to this, and it's often extremely quiet in its own way. You might notice in a sense that you're almost not breathing at all, and it shows that the breathing isn't associated with anything, including thought. This is a very interesting state, and it's a very calming state too.

You might notice with this as you begin to harmonize your breath, you might find out that you can easily get calm and your breath is easily stabilized and fine. You might notice this takes a few minutes, whereas in the beginning it might take you twenty minutes. As you continue to practice, you might start to notice that it only takes a moment or so to regulate your breath, and then you'll notice that your need to breathe out will start to grow less and less. You might notice that it even starts to vanish, and that you'll no longer be disturbed by anything.

You will notice by this point that your mind at this stage is very subtle, but also very calm. You might notice that while this trouble-free state is perfect, the way to it is often filled with many potholes, such as discomfort, restlessness, frustration, and even drowsiness.

If you start to notice that you're struggling with this, there are a few ways that you can work to make this easier on you, going from one to the next to help you become more skilled. You should in a relaxed manner do each of these exercises listed below and count each breath used in each exercise from 1-15.

- Start with the breaths, calling one cycle of exhaling and inhaling one breath
- Count only the inhaling you do
- Count only the exhaling that you do

Remember, as you reach fifteen, go back to one. As you get better with this, you might be able to count to a hundred or even more with this, without letting the mind wander or doping off because of how you're sitting. If you notice however that it is hard to not let your mind wander, or if you do doze off, you should start from the first step and begin all over once again. You will get frustrated, which is probably a natural human emotion and reaction to this, but as you get better, you'll find out that the breathing and your mind will become interdependent, and that confusion and sleepiness will increase as you start to have your breathing methods in all concentration, and your mind will become further calmed down.

Now that you know of the goals of breathing, it's time to apply this. You can do this with any meditation breathing, such as the beginner exercise later on. Your breathing is a huge part of this, and you'll notice as well the difference that this makes. You'll notice that your mind will also become calm and concentrated. By tracing your breath and regulating this, you'll have much more calmness, and much more concentration that will begin to depend as you feel your breath come and go. Notice as you do this how it leaves the pores as well. You might also notice in a sense that you're dissipating and melting away, and soon, you might feel a void in a sense. This is a strange sensation, because you might realize that you're free from everything, including illness and past situations that have held you back, and your mind reaches a level of quiet that you might not know before. You will then be able to trace your breath continuously.

Breathing gets you into a state of calmness, and this chapter is important for anyone working to master the art of breathing. It's something so simple that humans take for granted, but when you sit down and look at the mechanisms of breathing and what it all means, you'll begin to realize just how important it is to master this invaluable skill.

The mind is a very important part of this. With meditation, you can get many benefits from this as listed before, such as it can improve your health, increase your self-awareness, and give you energy, but the main goal here is to be free of thought. If you're free of thought, you'll be able to think with a mental clarity that you haven't before, and your true wisdom will shine through.

Now, we've discussed what to do with breathing. You will notice that counting the breath and tracing, you're regulating not only the breath, but also the mind. You'll notice that if you are concentrated in your entirety, your thoughts won't become a jumble of confusion, nor will they have an effect on you. Breathing and thought process are inherently connected, and it only takes one meditation session to realize this.

You might be someone who has racing mind or has emotional turmoil that continues to plague you. You might try this once, and if you do so, you'll see just how different it can change your entire thought process. Something so simple such as counting your breaths can change your entire outlook on your own personal thought processes. You might not even realize it until you do this, but once you do, you'll notice it changes everything.

With this, it will calm the mind, body, and also your breathing. When your body becomes more relaxed, you'll realize that you're free of the tension as well, and your breathing will start to slow down and deepen, which in turn will quiet down the mind and leave it undisturbed.

Now, as you continue in this, all of the finer points of the mind star to disappear. All of the disruptions and nuances start to change, and you'll start to realize that you'll need to control your mind, since it needs to become less erratic.

Now there are different ways to approach this, but the best way to do this is to have your attention on one point, and any thoughts that might arise are told to go away. This will start to change your thought process, because while your mind is calm, often the intrusive thoughts will come on in like uninvited guests, and you need to get rid of them.

Now, you don't have to be forceful with it, but instead you passively tell them to leave. You don't spend a ton of time on them either, taking less and less energy to look at each of them. You just tell them to go away after you acknowledge them.

If you get hung up on this, it'll lead to concentration, which isn't what you're going for. You want to make sure that you concentrate on one point of your choice, for it'll free you from the disturbing thoughts. With continued concentration will start to change the outlook of the practitioner, since they will start to notice that they have less disturbing thoughts coming through to them.

This can even extend as far as the entire day. If you for example, try this in the morning, you might start to notice that you have less attention on one of the areas of your life, but instead are in the here and now, and you're not disturbed by other such thoughts.

How to Do This

One way to improve your concentration is to figure out one point, and to focus on it. Now, the best thing to do is to make sure you pick something you're okay with looking at. You should concentrate and be relaxed about this. For example, some like to choose the tip of their nose, which is a great place to start. However, if you don't like the feeling of your eyes going a bit cross, you can choose your navel area or the point about an inch below it. You can use this to help restrict your mind from wandering, and some compare it to a monkey who has been running around willy-nilly suddenly restricted to a small space where you can't run and jump about. Now, you wouldn't do that to a monkey in real life, but if your mind is jumping around like a jumping bean, getting it to sit tight is probably one of the best things to do in order to regulate your thought.

Two Things to Plague You

When you're working to master your thought process, you'll start to notice how your mind changes. Meditation actually goes through both of these processes, and it's important to recognize, since many people just assume that you'll naturally improve your concentration, but that isn't the case.

The first things is when you sit down, you'll notice immediately that the mind is unstable, but also very restless. Your mind will try to pull you in every direction, trying to help you get through this in one moment, but then random tidbits you don't want to see will show up next, frustrating you.

You might start to notice that aches will come about as well, first in one area, and then anther. You might start to feel extreme discomfort, and you'll try to escape the pain and work to console the agony that you're going through. This isn't fun at all, and you'll try to imagine yourself somewhere else, doing something that isn't this in your life. You might even repeat important life events, something that you've had a great experience with. You might also start to realize you're dozing off too.

However, that's typically the first session, and the next step is that you'll notice that as you continue on, your mind will become more settled and your thoughts that are disturbing your mental clarity will diminish. There is still confusion there, and you'll still feel tired and doze off. At this point, start to sense the area about an inch below your navel. You will want to focus on that point, since it will help the disordered thoughts from impinging upon you, and it'll keep you from drifting off again and again, and it's a stabilizing effect that will improve your mental and physical health as well.

Now if you don't want to focus on that point, that's totally fine, it's not necessary. Figure out a point that works for you and simply focus on it, regardless of what it is.

Whatever you choose to get into, you will want to stay with this for the extent of the time that you've determined for sitting. For beginners, you should try to make this even more successful by making sure that you do this when you're most alert, and make sure to eliminate all of the distractions and discomforts that might be there so that you can have a better experience with this as well.

Insight Meditation

This is another type of concentration meditation, which differs from the one that you've been doing so far. For regular concentration meditation, if you have a distracting thought while concentrating, you immediately realize this and ignore the discriminating thought. It is a shallow way to get calm and avoid the thoughts that wander. If you do think about them, it'll just add a lot more to this that you shouldn't be doing. While concentrating might be great, you in essence want to do something completely different. You should instead focus on insight meditation.

Typically, you're always looking outside, at the external world, however with this approach, you want to put everything to the side, close your eyes, and in a sense observe, and from there feel the thoughts that are disrupting your thinking process. You can look at them, and from there, when you figure out that you can't actually hold onto them, you can simply send them away after this. Once you start to realize this, you begin to realize that you can dissolve and send this away. This is typically called original stillness and emptiness. When you develop this insight, you might reflect on the thought for a moment, but then it quickly disappears, replaced by an emptiness in there, which in turn creates a new way to make your mind work. It's pretty amazing, and mind-blowing. However, it requires you to have the ability to take the thought and throw it away. If you've done enough concentration meditation, you will be able to achieve this, but often, getting stuck in the distractive thoughts tends to happen, so master concentrative meditation before you begin with insight meditation.

You might think that thought will stop when you first meditate, but that isn't the case. You might actually realize that when you practice it for a while, it actually has increased. It's not necessarily the thought increasing, but it's more of the realization of what has been there all along, and the immediate source of suffering that you've been feeling is now apparent. You might have been blind to it for a long time, as many of us are, but in truth, once you see it, you'll start to realize just how enlightened that you are. You'll start to realize the truth of your existence.

Now, it's not totally abandoning the thought itself, but rather, you're working towards insights that have been there a long time, and that leads to the disappearance of this thought, and this actually is that stillness once more, of you've began to realize just what you've been missing, and the sudden enlightenment that you might start to realize over time.

With insight and concentration, you'll be able to improve your meditations all the more so. It's a deep process, and most of it is very mental, but if you realize this and work with it, it can actually help you quite a bit in your future understandings and endeavors.

Now, mindfulness meditation is something that you might not normally practice. However, it's definitely something that can change your thought process. This chapter will go into further detail on mindfulness, and why we need mindfulness meditation.

A Society that Takes Everything for Granted

For many of us, we take our lives for granted. From walking, to driving, to even the foods that we eat, we're not totally in tune with what we're doing. That might seem like no big deal, but you're actually missing out on some valuable insight because of that, and often, it leaves us in a mental fog that won't let us actually realize the potential that we've got.

When we drive or do other sorts of actions, we tend to go on automatic. That means we'll do it, but we won't pay attention. Accidents happen because of this, and often, we end up not realizing just how important something is until it's too late. We're not mindful of our actions, and because of that, we tend to not realize what we're doing at all.

However, we can start to actually be mindful of our actions, becoming better observers because of it. We can pay more attention to our surroundings, and not take as much for granted. Who knows, you might not even realize just how much you've taken for granted until you've sat back and realized it. That's where mindfulness meditation comes on in, and it's important to have a sense of mindfulness when you're looking into bettering yourself, and participating in this.

With mindfulness, you'll become more observant of what your area looks like. You'll be able to be there without problems or disruptive thoughts, and overall, you'll be much happier. People use this type of thought process to help better themselves, and be more grateful for their actions in life.

Mindfulness in meditation

Now remember that every moment gives you a chance to meditate, which is why you should consider mindfulness. However, with our daily lives, we feel that we're too busy, or that we can't just up and do it, because we require structure. In that case, if you feel like you can't spend copious amounts of time doing this, you should set up some time either during your meditations, or at another point, and start to work on your mindfulness. Some people love to do it first thing in the morning or before bed, but whenever you do it is based on you.

Ideally, you should try to do this multiple times a day, but if you can only do it once a day due to time constraints, figure out when is best for you, especially with the availability that you have, and also your own personal responsiveness. You shouldn't do this when you're tired, that's for sure. You should look for the quality in the time that you put aside, rather than the quantity of your time spent doing this.

When you're doing this, you should regard this as a time to unwind or rest, or some form of relaxation. What you should do is try to do this, not spending it doing anything at all, and not a time to be engaged in anything. Just give yourself some time to relax. At this point, it might even be hard for you here, since at the onset, it might actually be something almost foreign to you, but you should then practice it naturally, rather than trying to do so through an act of your own determination or the like. You want to do it when it feels most natural. For example, you might only want to spend about ten minutes a day doing this, since you don't have the time to be that mindful.

However, you might end up extending it for a minute each and every day. You might want to do it another minute later on. Finally, after a while, you're sitting for almost an hour at a time, and you'll be able to really just sit there each day. You want to form a habit with this, since we are in essence creatures that love habits. You should also make sure that the place will be unperturbed each day, since often, many people tend to get annoyed if things don't act like this.

You can actually try this form of meditation while you're in bed as well, not even leaving the area. To do this, you should wake up, and when you're becoming more aware, you should put your palms over your solar plexus and then move them slowly down your lower abdomen. You should proceed to do this several times, being mindful of your entire hand placement. You can then get up and head to the bathroom and get ready for the day. Do this right before you sit down and practice if you do so first thing in the morning.

You can do this other times of the day as well if you have a natural time for yourself that you do your meditations. It soon becomes natural to breathe like this, which is a great way to get yourself in tune with your body. This is helpful for many, since more often than not, people aren't even mindful of their chest area, and even just letting your palms move down can certainly help you acknowledge this.

However, it is more than just a natural routine, it's actually an experience. You should take this time as a time to discover who you are, through relaxation and observation in a passive manner. You don't even need to spend a time of time on this, but rather just a couple of moments observing the state of your body. You'll realize the amazing difference that this makes when you're doing this, and it can be the most refreshing feeling when you know you'll have a busy day.

Mindful Eating

Another way that you can use it is with eating. For many of us, we never think about the food that we put in our mouth, but rather we just eat it. However, you can actually use food as a form of meditation in a sense. It might seem a bit silly. After all, we always think about the food we're eating, right? But do you ever just sit there actually eating your food, thinking about the food and not actually thinking about the five hundred other things you need to do that day? Chances are, as soon as you sit down, this will actually make you realize that you won't do that. However, you'll certainly realize right then and there that you definitely need to work on this, since it's something that you'll definitely realize you don't do. It can be a very trying experience, and the simple practice actually brings about a whole slew of disruptive thoughts. You might realize that there are feelings of deprivation there, along with anxiety that you normally don't feel before. If you're the type of person who typically looks at your phone or other sources while eating, you might realize that this is super hard since it actually involves you leaving that crutch. However, the purpose of this isn't to make you feel bad, but rather, it's to show you that you're relying on these attachments far more than you care to believe. You might also realize the natural inclination to be a part of it, and once you realize that awareness and need, you'll be able to alleviate yourself of this. It's a mind-blowing experience, and it can change your life. Below are the steps to do it, and you'll soon be able to avail yourself of these amazing benefits that you could obtain from this.

Now how to do mindful eating is simple. First of all, you shouldn't eat before you meditate, since it does make some sleepy. If you end up overeating as well, you might be distracted by the fullness. If you don't eat before you sit it also can hurt you too, since you might feel weak, suffer from headaches, and your breathing might be thrown off. In essence, you should eat about thirty or so minutes before, listening to the needs that you have.

When you do eat, pay attention to what you're eating the entire time. You should feel the texture of the food as it hits your mouth, the clank of the utensils, whatever it might be. You should become mindful of your chewing, and also how much you are eating. If you do this before you sit, it gets you into the mindset of meditation in a much better manner.

For some of us, we might realize we actually eat way more than we should. For many of us, the reason why we might be overweight, have issues with our health, and the like, might not even be because of something complicated but rather, it's not being mindful of how much you're eating. This exercise will allow you to realize just how much you're eating, and you can take the necessary actions to really help yourself if you feel like you're eating too much.

Now for some that engage in this, it can be almost miraculous as well. Your life might end up feeling more orderly, since you're not involving yourself in spending all this time eating anymore, and you might notice that since you've stopped overeating, you might be losing weight. This definitely can be a big observation, and you might as well notice other sorts of symptoms as well.

You might realize that you have other symptoms as well when you're being mindful of eating. You can feel unrest, headaches, symptoms of depression and anxiety, stomach troubles, clouded thinking, itching, and even fatigue if you start mindfully eating. However, the best thing to do if you do notice this is to find out what the cause of this is, and also start to get rid of the symptoms.

For those that suffer addiction to food, this can be much harder, since often these are the characteristics of this, and for those that have allergies to food, it can also be caused by this. However, instead of focusing on the symptoms, you find the root cause of this, passively aware of what is going on, and from there you will end up relaxing. This will not only help with any reactions you get to food, but you might even know what is troubling you. Because of this awareness of what happened, you won't want to act on it, and you'll start to feel a sense of liberation.

In essence, you want to find out what is best for you. You should listen to your body and become mindful of what you're eating, how you're eating, and the like. This is the same with when you should meditate. Some like to do it an hour after a meal, or maybe thirty minutes. For this, you're wanting to observe, and once you discover these points, you'll be able to push them away passively, and you'll be more aware of what is happening all the time because of this.

Mindful Sleeping

This can even be applied to sleeping. For many people, we often take sleep for granted. Yes, it is a major part of our routines in life, and we need sleep. If you don't sleep for a few days, your body will begin to shut down. Some people believe that their sleep is almost robotic though, and often some might miss a night or two just to stay awake, but often, it muddles a person's concentration and it makes it harder to work as well. However, for some, sleeping too much can make you feel sluggish as well.

Becoming mindful of your sleeping and how it affects you is a big part. Pay attention to your body as you go off into sleep, using a deep breath each and every moment. You should feel your body relax, and you'll feel it almost in a dreamlike state. When you sleep, if you actually pay mind to relax, you'll realize how different it makes you. Some people sleep for the sake of sleeping, since they need it to function, but if you actually realize what sleep can do for you, you'll begin to realize how amazing it is, and how you need to have it.

Some people also need to pay mind to their body's awake hours. For some, going to bed at two in the morning and getting up at ten is the best thing for them, for maybe they're programmed to work more at night. For some, going to bed at ten or so and getting up at six is the best means, because they work on an early riser schedule.

If you wake up at night and you realize that you're not sleepy or struggle to fall asleep, you actually can use meditation here. You can simply sit and become mindful of the sights and sounds there using your breathing in order to really feel every single movement and motion in the environment. You will feel your body relax, and before you know it, you'll begin to feel yourself grow sleepier as well. This might take a few minutes off of sleeping, but it's better than being restless. You can become mindful as well of whatever restlessness is happening to you, so that you can do away with it accordingly. Whatever works for you, do try to use it, since it can make everything much easier for you.

For some, it even gets to the point where they don't really need a ton of sleep, but instead use meditation instead. While this isn't something for everyone, and you should listen to your body, you should take the time to acknowledge that you might just need less sleep. Your body has become more mindful of the environment and atmosphere, so making sure that you listen and realize it's developing naturally can aid you in the understanding of your body.

Environmentally Mindful

Finally, become more mindful of the environment. You should sit or walk around a place, and become more mindful of the people around here. Maybe look at the people, acknowledge them, see what they are doing, whatever it might be. If you find your thoughts getting away from the present moment, you can always bring them back to where they belong. This is a very important type of meditation if you really want to be in the moment, experiencing it all, and making sure that you're fully aware.

This is a great technique to use before you're driving. Five minutes before, sit in the car, and become mindful of your environment. Become mindful of the controls, of where your foot is on the floor, of the feel of the seats, of the way the interior looks, of the environment around. Just become aware. If you feel a distracting thought coming about, you can push it away, and you'll begin to realize just what you haven't noticed before. Car accidents and the like are often caused by people not paying enough attention to the area around them, and it's often a major problem. However, if you become more mindful of everything, you'll see for yourself just how different everything looks, and how you've been missing out on quite a bit of the world around yourself.

Mindfulness sis a very important part of meditation. We take life for granted, however, if we spend the time to look at the area around us, becoming mindful of our body and the relation to the environment, we'll begin to learn the difference that this makes ultimately. It can change your life for the better, and it can make it even more amazing as well. Do this for yourself, and see the difference that it makes when it comes to viewing the world from a different sort of lens.

There is another form of meditation that many people often don't think about when they're thinking of meditation. This is movement meditation, and it's often one that many people who are energetic and want to become mindful of their movements engage in. It's pretty mind-blowing just what it can do for you, and this chapter will go over what it is, and how to get the most results from it, including some key concepts to keep in mind.

What is it?

Movement meditation is a lot less complicated than you think. Essentially, it's meditation where you move. This involves a range of techniques, and it was touched upon in a previous chapter, but there is more to that hasn't been explored. In essence, this is great for those who have energy, and it can even have mindfulness applied if you do it at a slow speed.

Now, the best time to do this is when we're energetic. If we're trying our hardest to sit, often that can be counterproductive, so why would you waste your time doing it. It actually is better to move around, since it can often help with this extra energy. It needs to go somewhere, so movement meditation is ideal for it.

Many monasteries use this too. It isn't just something that a few do. It can be used in tandem with sitting if you want to alternate them, and you typically walk in order to give the body a bit of exercise to help get rid of the excess energy, and also to help with physical tension that is stuck there.

Now, our bodies are a part of the spiritual path of understanding ourselves. Now, while the mind is usually what we think about in meditation, the body is a tool that can really help with this as well. In most types of meditation, mind is what you focus on, and often emotions are there too. However, the body is also a major factor.

The body can be a part of the exploration, and it does give you a path. Some consider the body to be the enemy, but in essence, the body is actually a means to do what we want mentally. We should work to improve our body because in turn, we can further improve our spiritual nature and even the state of our body as well.

Remember, the body doesn't need to have concepts to it, like the mind typically does. So, when we observe something directly, we're already in the non-conceptual stage which is often what takes a while for sitting meditation. The body is also a part of the physical universe, so meditation will help us understand the world itself, and even the relationship of our body to the rest of the world out there.

The body isn't some illusion or anything either. Often, people try to claim the body is a defiled sort of structure, but in essence, it's how the soul connects to the world itself. We can learn about the nature of life through the body as well. The world is always changing, moving, interacting with life through the body as well, and since the body is in motion constantly, this constantly-moving particle is in relationship to other moving particles, which in essence, gives one a deeper connection.

Slower movements in meditation often create a calmer mind, and that is the goal of meditation. While you might think moving about fast will help with the excess energy, we're often not mindful of it, so we won't make great spiritual progress. Instead you want to focus on having slow and steady movements, for it can make a difference in your body and how it reacts to the rest of the world.

Guidelines for Movement Meditation

There are a few guidelines to this, and you should keep them in mind. They aren't forced, but in order to get the most results from this form of meditation, it's advised that you partake in this.

- Become mindful of everything: you want to be mindful of the motions that you're making with the muscles, how we contact various surfaces, such as our hands touching various objects or even the floor, the movement of the energies within the body in relation to the outside world, the natural responses to stimuli that are out there, such as music, the position of our body parts in this space, the sensations you might feel such as pressure and pain, your breathing and how it sounds, whether or not it's right breathing or deep breathing, and the state of the stillness that exists in every single activity out there. You want to be mindful of all of this. This might sound way harder than it is, but once you get the hang of it, it'll be better.

- Focus on all parts of the body. While some types of movement meditation might focus on one part, such as maybe a yoga pose loosening some sort of muscles in the body, most forms of meditation want you to be attentive to everything. If it calls for you to be attentive to muscles, you can be, but you don't need to be, but rather look at the bigger picture. You should try to notice things that you normally ignore, such as maybe your fingertips, toes, the tip of your nose, or even maybe the way you stand and hold yourself. You might not even be aware of this. With every single movement, you should focus on every single part and actually look at the state, since you might not realize that some parts are in a certain state. Think of your belly button. It's actually numb, and you might not like it, since it's not what you see. You should look for every single one of these parts, and instead of throwing them to the side, start to give them love and acceptance, and even tell them to join you once again, and you can feel a visualization of this body part coming back to your body, functioning in a general manner. Now all of this is often done in a mental state, but you might feel some physical side effects from this as well.

- There if often this misunderstanding that the body is our own and we own it. In a sense, it is a living organism in it of itself, with its own consciousness and needs, especially if you think on a cellular level. If you think about the body sensations, the vitality, the chemical actions in there, your breathing, your body temperature, and even your movements, you'll be able to start to realize how different and distanced you were from this. You might start to realize that you are actually not seeing the body as an entity, and often, this can shock you.

- Let the body move on its own. You want to let the body do what it wants to. You can try this by leaning to the left and then having the body rigid with the muscles completely tight. Then, go back to the upright position, and then, try this next step. Think about leaning, begin the motion, but then let the body lean in its own way, doing this slowly. You will notice that the body is controlling this movement, and that can change the insight that you typically have with it. You might notice the adjustments of every muscle and even the internal tissues. You might notice the pauses and rhythms of the body that are used. You might notice that you are seeking pleasure with every movement, and you might even notice the changes in breathing and the exertion that is used. Simply letting the body move will provide you with a mindfulness of all of this.

- You will want to move slowly. This will allow us to look at the motions within a larger motion. Often, we move very fast. Our bodies are constantly in this rushed state, and we don't even notice our muscles moving in each movement. However, take your arm and raise it super-fast. Then raise it slowly. You will notice the various events going on in the body. You might take as long as about thirty seconds to a minute to move your arm completely straight up since it's mindful of that motion. There are various muscles that can be used in each of these, the joints changing, and even a balancing of the body from this, and a heat that is pushed into the muscles, along with the stretching of the tissue to improve the movement of the arms. This is done very slowly, since you want to make sure that you account for all of the bodily motions. Whether the motion is with the hands and the feet, keep this in mind.

- Have the motions as the forefront rather than the goal. You shouldn't be thinking about where you're going, but instead think of the motions.
- Finally, have a lightness. When your body moves at its own pace, you'll start to feel a lightness of your own movements, a sort of effortlessness that goes along with it. You should let the body naturally move you easily, and then, you should let it move in its own regard to help with the vitality of this.

With these concepts, keep them in mind, for they can make a difference in your overall goal of understanding the relationship of the body with other parts, and it can make understanding all the easier.

Movement Meditation Techniques

Now while you don't have to follow a set guideline to it, there are a few techniques that you can use to get the most from movement meditation. This section will go over what they are, and what each of them consists of, and how to get the best results from each.

First, move with every single motion in tandem with the way you breathe. When you breathe, do so at a natural rate, which is a controlled speed. You can walk with this, or whatever movement that you want to do with your body.

Then, take your palms and put them on your chest. When you inhale in, move the arms out in front of you, and when you exhale, you should bring them back to your chest. You will notice with this that there is an energy from the breath alone that is pushing the arms outward and breathing them back. Become mindful of the relationship between this and your arm movements.

Next, you can sit down, and from there, slowly stand up. However, you want to do this extremely slowly, noticing in a sense that your body is growing in length in a sense, such as your neck going upward, the back longer, and soon, the entire body is in a standing position. You can then walk forward, and you will notice with every single step the lengthen of your legs as you do push each of these forward. Do this for a couple of minutes, and then go back to where you were sitting and do the same thing.

Next, if you want to try this, you can begin from standing or sitting. Focus on moving the spine and the rest of yourself in very subtle motions. You are looking to have the perfect posture, one that is both relaxing and comfortable for every single part of you. With this, you can scan the body for any discomfort in various area, and from there change your position until your body is in the ideal position. This can be a great means to help fix any posture and sitting issues that you might have.

If you want to, you can then take your two, and then spend about twenty seconds looking at each joint and moving it slowly back and forth. You should start with the big toe and then work your way to the end. You should do both sides, and you should notice the sensations with every single joint in a vivid manner.

You can also try synchronizing the rhythm of your movements with your heartbeat. This is a bit of a harder one to try, but it ultimately can be very rewarding. What you want to do is to first, listen to your heartbeat, become mindful of it. Then, slowly extend your arm and start to let it move to your side. You can even do this in tandem with walking if you so desire. Begin to explore this, looking at each and every single precise movement as you go along. For many, this can be quite hard, but if you take a simple motion to synchronize, it's much easier.

Finally, work to experiment with the varying degrees of supervision that you might have when you're controlling the movements of your body. You might realize that you're not letting the body do what it wants to, and from there, it can actually change your entire outlook. Instead, you should start to balance this out between what the body wants, and the mind's control, and you can do this easily. To begin, you should try it with raising your arm straight up.

When you do this at first, you should do it willfully, having your muscles nice and tight. You should then, when it comes back down, do it this time in a relaxed manner, keeping the feedback there such as your comfort and discomfort, and then respond to this by moving in a natural manner.

On the last time, you should simply intend that the arm will go up, and then, with a very gentle will, nothing too strong, simply let your arm move upwards, almost floating and such, and then, let the arm start to get creative with itself. Let the upper arm, forearm, the hands and fingers start to find their way there. They might not do it in a rigid manner, but instead, they might even twist and bend, almost like a paper bag flying in a breeze. This might be a bit strange to you, but you might start to notice that it's almost like a dance for you, with every single subtle movement occurring from the body's own expressions and their own sense of pleasure. You actually won't even notice the self-conscious there, and often, this allows a much freer state of movements.

We tend to take our motions for granted, and in many cases, we don't even truly know our body as much as we think we do. But we end to let the body move on the will of the mind, nothing more, however, sometimes the ultimate solution to this isn't just letting the mind control everything, but to let the body control its own state, and its own future. If you've felt a sense of mindlessness when you think about the body, try this. It's a form of meditation that will allow you to increase your own heightened sense of spirituality, and allow the connection between yourself, and your body, to become that much stronger as well.

For many people, they expect to have these results come immediately. With meditation, they think that one session is often all that it takes, and for many, that's why they give up when they don't get a result after their first sitting. However, it's important to go into the finer details of what is going on when you meditate, and why you shouldn't try to work towards results the entire time, but instead, just let the natural state come to you.

Perseverance and Results

Now, the biggest hurdle that beginners in meditation start to realize, is that it can be very uncomfortable to begin with. This is why many people abandon meditation when they take it on, because they realize that it isn't easy. The practice of sitting in the position, focusing on breathing and mindfulness, can be overwhelming, however, there is a way to get past this.

While some might feel like this even when they're not beginners, the biggest thing to remember is that perseverance is the answer to everything. You might not want to go on, simply because the idea of sitting for another five minutes will drive you insane, but if you think about it, that's just an intrusive thought. You're just letting the intrusive thoughts win if you do that, and often, if you do give into that, you won't get better.

How you get better is perseverance. You need to make progress simply by perseverance, and you can sit there every single day at the same time in the same place, and you just want to become aware of what is going on, having a light concentration, and free of the distractive thoughts. It might take you weeks, even months, before you feel a big change, but often, when it happens, it's life-changing. You might even realize just how big it is until you sit there and think about it, and soon, life has a different meaning. Often, you just have to work at it, and the results will show up.

Speaking of results, don't look for them. Don't go into this with the forced idea that you need to have results. Here's the thing, like with everything, if you're going into this forcefully looking for results, you won't get anywhere with it. That is the harsh truth. When you're meditating, you will start to realize that as you go along, the thought will fall away, and soon, you'll start to realize that a natural state of mind is there. That is the healthy mindset that you're going for, since it's free of desire and the stresses of this.

If you go into this with the idea that you have to have this goal, almost forcefully in a sense, you won't get anywhere. That's a disruptive thought, and you need to do away with these disruptive thoughts. This is something that many who begin with meditation struggle with quite often. It's hard to just let go and let your body and mind relax, getting rid of all thought.

The idea of having no aim is a hard concept for those to understand. In life, we're always moving towards a goal, always moving towards a higher purpose, and that higher purpose is so ingrained in our minds that it often becomes obsessive. We have to get there, we have to achieve this goal, we have to do this, we have to do that. All too often, that is actually a very unhealthy mindset, and if you start to realize that you're obsessive over your goals, it can change you.

With meditation, the goal is to not have a goal. Don't have some forced need for results. This is very misunderstood by many, and it's hard for many to grasp. Our obsessions to succeed and excel are what push us forward, and to just get rid of these inclinations is often almost unreal to many of us. The key reason why though, is because it breaks the illusion of control.

Control is something we also obsess over. Typically, if you're obsessive over having results, it's because you have a fixed control over this. It's an illusion that you've put forward, and when you start to realize that you don't have to control everything, it can be quite scary. But all too often, it can change your life, and it can show you a new meaning that you've never understood before. It's scary, yes, but often, understanding this point can change the mindset that you've had, and the future that you've put forward, allowing you to fully feel the state of relaxation that meditation tries to purport.

Don't Have Concern

Another big thing that people tend to obsess over are their own concerns and cares. With the stress of life, it can often be almost overwhelming to get rid of these. We tend to stress and care about many things, but often, that actually is holding us back. Have you ever just abandoned all cares, and instead just worked on being in the moment? It can be quite hard, but it actually is a way to change you. You shouldn't have obsessive cares at the forefront when you're meditating, but instead, work on your breathing and your mind. If you start to feel those cares come forward, they will come and go. If you don't care about them, you'll start to realize just how calm everything is, and how your mind becomes calmer.

If you close your eyes while you sit, you might not see the outside things. The sounds might be there, but you will start to realize that they are actually still disturbing. You might also feel those inner thoughts and concerns start to crop up. This might be a bit disturbing for many, and this can be quite cumbersome, but if you start to throw away those cares, it will take you to a certain moment, a moment that will utterly change you.

In that specific moment, if you start to realize that you are aware of what you're doing, and that those problems are just problems, you can drop them away. You'll start to realize that those sounds are just that, sounds. They don't need to be combed over or anything. Rather, you don't have to focus on them, but instead, focus on being there and just completely observing. That is the goal.

If your life is riddled with concerns, just go meditate. Don't let those concerns beat you, but instead you should just acknowledge them as they do along, and then drop them.

Physical Manifestations and Meditation

For some, another big problem that they run into is physical manifestations. Often, when people are forcefully expecting results and the like, they often start to feel various symptoms. Even when you're just sitting there and experiencing, this can ultimately happen, and this can deter one's perseverance. However, if this does happen, don't let it get the best of you.

Some people get very hot, overly sweaty, start to have violent shaking, hearing various sounds, and some might even start to see things or do various positions they weren't even thinking about doing. If you start to notice this, don't suppress the manifestations. Most people don't actually have this, but often struggle with the intrusive thoughts, but instead, you want to keep on practicing. This is often a manifestation of just sitting there inside the moment, and while it is scary, by doing so, you'll end up feeling much better health as well.

Sometimes, various habits that you might have will start to come up. You might feel the need to obsessively bite your nails, your lips, or whatever. If this does happen, recognize that this is a manifestation of the training, and don't be alarmed. You should work through this, and often, if you're struggling, this is the way to get the benefits of this.

One might say that this is karma, but often it's not really the case. It's something that can be a symptom of the factors of meditation, and you might start to feel other various mental and physical symptoms. If you start to feel these and you start to get upset, you should just undemand that the void you might end up feeling is there, and it changes constantly. Nothing is real because nothing has inherent nature, so if there is nothing, you don't have to crave or reject it. This is a bit of a profound viewpoint, but often, this can be a way to understand how to overcome these factors.

However, if you start to give into these, giving up every single time that you do suffer from these problems, it will only trap you. You won't ever get better, and it's important to understand that you need to work through this. The way to get out of the state that you're in is to get through it, and while most people don't feel this when meditating, you might end up suffering from some aches and pains. Don't let it best you, and don't give up, but instead, get through it.

With meditation, understanding that various actions can come up, including the need to have an obsessive result, can hold you back. By looking at this, realizing what is truly going on and changing yourself for the better, you'll feel much better about this, and ultimately, you'll have a much stronger sense of control as a result.

Chapter 12: How to Regulate your body, breathing, movement, and mind

Now for everyday practice, it's important to realize that the body, mind, and your breathing are interdependent and sometimes they are seen as the same aspects of the same thing in some ways. In Buddhism, there are practices that help you control these aspects, and where are methods that you can use to help you get through your practices. These methods that you're about to learn can actually help you get in and get out of meditation.

Now, your everyday activities are something you should first think about. If you are doing anything with a roughness to it, that will change your breathing. It'll become rough as well. If your breathing becomes rough, your mind will become rough and muddled, and when you do sit, you might feel uneasy and almost confused as well.

Now not everyone has a life that is easy to really do in a gentle manner. The hustle and bustle of the office, of heavy labor, and the like can make. One way is to visualize yourself as being relaxed and sitting when you do sit down to practice. Actually have that mindset when you do so, and just think about it. You should do this before you begin. It's a very simple procedure, and you'll notice that you do feel warm and relaxed, and you can then perfect your sitting position to make it more fitting for yourself. Try that, for it can help you with ensuring that your body does have the best position and state for meditation.

Now for the body, it was mentioned before how you want to sit, but if you're often struggling with pain from sting on the surface, find one that best fits you. Remember, comfort is what you're going for. If you have cushions, bring them over to help support the body.

You should then get yourself in the half-lotus position, or in the Indian style position if you are still unable to get there completely. However, you should try to go for lotus, since it often yields the best results when it comes to getting the best responses from meditation.

If you want to do the full lotus you certainly can as well. However, it is a bit more complicated.

Now if you don't know how to do a half-lotus, that's okay. It's simple. You should sit in an upright position with the knees on each side and the legs crossed near the ankle area. You should then take the left limb that is lower and put it on top of the right thigh and then slide the left leg in close to where your lower belly is, so that you can have the left sole turned upwards and the toes of the left foot are parallel to where your thigh is. You should make sure that they're all parallel before you begin.

If you want full lotus, you can start by putting your right lower leg on the left, and then turn the right sole up and bring it close to where your lower belly is. When it's done, if you're wearing a belt, make sure to loosen it so that you can have it not slip off, and make sure that you have anything else that is binding off of yourself as well. If your collar is tight, loosen it, if your watch is digging in, take care of that, if your bra is tight, undo the clasp. When you're done, take the back of your left palm and put it upright, and then rest the right hand in the same way. Put them both on your feet. You can then check your posture, to see if there is any leaning, strain on your body, and slumping, and adjust yourself as needed.

If your limbs are still super tight, or if you've checked that there is any straining, start to shake the limbs a few times gently in order to relax them. You should then check to see how you are sitting. Don't be slumped down, but make sure that you have correct posture and are erect as well.

Remember to not have the head forward or leaning, and your chin shouldn't be pulled in. It should be a natural sit. You can then start to exhale from your mouth to get all of the extra air that is out. You should then close your lip so that everything is tight, and then close your eyes. Breathe in through your nose, and soon, start to sit and meditate. This will help prevent any slacking that could happen.

Regulating Breath

Now it was touched on before how important it is to have a regulated breath. If you start to realize that you are breathing in an audible fashion, it's actually disruptive. A gasping breath and a coarse one is also disruptive too, and you should work to get to a restful one. A restful breath is barely noticed, and it's so fine that most people don't even realize that you're breathing, and it also causes comfort and ease.

Now, when you are sitting, you should breathe until you get restful. You will want to make sure that you're persistent with this. If you start to notice that it's not fine, that means that it's not regulated, so keep on going. If you get upset, don't despair, but instead, just continue on trying, and continue to breathe.

Remember as well, that when you're concentrating right, you will grow relaxed. As you start to relax more and you're concentrating in a thoughtful manner, you'll relax way more than before. You will then start to breathe as well in a more restful manner.

With breathing as well, don't expect it to be just through your nose. It's actually a full-body sort of experience. You can practically imagine the feeling of breathing through all of your pores as you do this, and while it might seem strange now, it can really help you if you're trying to fully understand the extent of your breathing, and to help you regulate your breathing in a fast manner.

Regulating the Mind

With the mind in meditation, the goal is to get rid of confusion and thinking, and to help with wandering attention, and to help stabilize the mind when it starts to diffuse, sink, float, or even become strained. Often, a sinking mind is dull and confused, with some dozing as well. If you start to notice this, you should then start to put your attention to the tip of your nose.

If you notice that your mind is floating, it starts to drift, and you might begin to feel almost uneasy and not really concerned about what is going on. If that is the case, you will want to make sure that you do fix your attention as well, since it'll keep the thoughts from coming up. When that is done, the mind will soon start to stabilize and it will calm down. By having that slight focal point, you can then regulate the mind. Typically, these steps happen when you enter meditation.

Now sustained meditation is the next step. When you have wariness without intention, you will want to keep this. You want to be constantly aware of what your body, breathing and your mind are doing. Once you've regulated the body and sat for a bit, and have also regulated the mind as well, you might notice that everything is becoming a bit loose and strained, or maybe you're moving to a side, drooping, holding your shoulders in a strained manner, you will want to adjust this. This might happen if you do this for a duration, and while it is correctable, it isn't what you should be going for. You want to go back and start to regulate everything there, making sure that everything is together.

For some though, it actually might end up being a bit of an interesting situation. The body might be regulated, but the breathing isn't, and even when you've focused on that, it might take a bit to get it all together. You might notice that while the breathing and the body are regulated, your mind isn't. You should then start to regulate the mind once more. With meditation, it can cause you to lose a bit of control of your three factors. However, your goal is to have all of these working together in tandem with one another. For some, they might not have trouble with this, but for others, it can be a struggle. You should use these in whatever order you need to, not in succession, since it might be only one part that is out of sorts. You might need a bit of time to understand this, and it's kind of like learning how to ride a bike. Once you do so, it's all natural.

The goal of meditation is really to sustain all of this, and essentially, that's what you want to go for when you're working on every single one of these. Have all three of these working together in a harmonious fashion, and you'll start to notice for yourself the difference that this makes ultimately in terms of what this could mean for you.

Now, the final part of this is learning how to come out of meditation, and getting your mind back to where it needs to be. You should before the session is over use your mouth to inhale and exhale, visualizing the air starting to leave these various parts of yourself. You might notice how tense you might be when you start to move. You should start to rotate your shoulders, arms, extremities, neck and head, and start to relax everything. You might not notice just how much of the feeling in your body left when you start to do this.

Once you're done, start to rub your body with your hands, making sure to feel every single part of it, and then start to take your palms, rubbing them together, then gently over your eyes, holding them there for a moment. When you've started to feel like everything is back to normal, and you've cooled down, you can slowly start to get up. It might take a second to really move, simply because it often causes the feeling of the body to leave for a moment, but once you do gain feeling back, you can leave the area you were sitting in.

Now when you do this, you don't want to be too fast with this, especially since this can cause you to destabilize. If that happens, there might be headaches and illnesses that can erupt, and it often isn't what you should be doing. Take it slow.

Tips for a Distracted Mind

Now for some, even if they do try, their mind is coarse and unsettled. Now, for some, it can also be them obsessively looking at various things, such as maybe sexual desire, whether it be in a positive or negative manner, this can often cause you to be distracted and take you out of meditation. This is another thing to regulate, and while it isn't encouraged to be done all the time, you should definitely do this if you start to notice that you're getting overwhelmed by this.

To do this, if you start to notice that you're in a sexual desire, with an opposite view, or maybe some sort of anger, you can instead get out of this by working to express compassion otherwise. The opposite of this will cause you to see that this is an illusion, and if you notice this, you'll start to be able to bring yourself back. If you do notice this, throw some compassionate this, and once you do this, you'll be able to halt any sort of discrimination that might be coming about.

If you start to notice that you're not really looking into things, but they are overwhelming your mind, you can do this as well. You should look at the nature of things, noticing that they don't have an inherent existence, and that the apparent cycle is dependent on the causes, which in turn are dependent on the experiences of the past and in the present circumstances. From this, you can extrapolate that cause doesn't have an inherent nature, and that they're identical with an undifferentiated reality that they come from. If you notice that they are unreal, you'll be able to make them go away, so they will cease to arise.

This is good if you start to meditate and you realize you're stuck in some sort of moment, whether it be a traumatic moment of the past or the like. If that is the case, you should make sure that you take the time to fully understand this, realizing that it isn't real, that nothing is real, and you can do away with the thought that is there.

Controlling the mind, body, and your breathing is the way to get the most results from meditation. By taking the time to fully explore every single one of these, you'll be able to fully understand the meaning of this practice, and it will make your life and every part of this understanding much easier to bear.

For many who begin, they need something that will get them fully set up to meditate. These ten steps are the simplest ways to begin, and you can read each of them as you go along. If you want a quick and dirty means to meditate, then this is the one for you. This is typically under the umbrella of sitting meditation as well.

1) Find a place where you can sit tall. Often, the best way to begin meditation is to sit. You should sit either on the floor, in a chair, or even on a stool if that's comfy. If you're on the floor, cross your legs. You want to be comfortable, but you also don't want to slouch. You should feel almost as if you're a puppet, being pulled by a string and extending your head and neck area, allowing you to sit up in a straight line. For those that tend to slouch, this can

be quite the first step, but if you master this then you're well on your way.

2) Your next step is to relax. You can do this either via closing your eyes and scanning your body from the bottom of it all the way to the top, and letting each part rest at a time, or do it with your eyes partially open, but still scanning and relaxing every single part. With many people, it can be hard to do this with their eyes closed, so work with what works for you.

3) The next step is to be silent and keep yourself still. This is much harder than you might think, especially if you're prone to restlessness. However, you want to just be still and sit. Become aware of what is around you, such as the sounds you might hear, your surroundings, and even your body. You should acknowledge them and be aware, but don't get up

to change them. If you hear a bird, just be aware that there is a bird. Don't focus on it.

4) You will also want to focus on your breathing once you've mastered the art of sitting there and keeping yourself still. You want to pay attention to your breathing, but don't obsessively focus on this. You want to take slow, deep breaths. You will want to have your diaphragm engaged and fill your lungs up, but make sure that your breath isn't forced. You want to also make sure that you breathe through your nose and out through your mouth, for it will give you the most engaged, relaxed breath, and it will allow you to fully acknowledge what your breathing is doing.

5) The next part, which you don't need to have, but for some it is encouraged, is a mantra. These are not something complicated, but instead they are a sound, a phrase you might use, or even a single word

that you say throughout the duration of the meditation. They can have really good spiritual benefits, and it can even be transformative and vibrational as well. They allow you to have a focal point during meditation if you so need one. You can say these either out loud or at yourself, and they are definitely worth it if you're struggling with this. If you want to do this, you can start with "om" or even "I am breathing in, I am breathing out." Don't force the words, but just naturally say them.

6) Next, you will want to calm your mind. This comes with the breathing and the mantra, whichever you prefer to use. Typically, you will start to notice this, but this also doesn't mean that the thoughts won't go away. You will still get thoughts from this, and you can simply acknowledge them and more on when they come forward, and you should pay attention to the mantra or breathing. You shouldn't

put your entire focus on your thoughts. Some days, this might start to become much harder than others, but other days, it's super easy, so you need to remember that both parts of the spectrum will happen, but you shouldn't dwell on this. You shouldn't focus on anything that is from the outside, but instead, just let it be, and then move on.

7) For this, you choose how long you want to do this. With this type of meditation, and really any meditation period, there isn't any sort of delineated time. You should probably start with about 5-10 minutes or so, and as you start to grow more comfortable, focusing on practicing longer. If you need to, especially if you've been sitting for a long time, need something to get you out of this, you can set an alarm to let you know when you're done. You typically shouldn't be doing this for hours, unless of course, you really want to. For some people, you can

actually couldn't your breathing and when you've hit a certain number of breaths, you can end it. However, this method does tend to fail, because you'll be much more focused on the number instead of just being there.

8) When you are done, the next phase is to bring your attention back to where you are, seeing the space and presence around you. You should then start to wiggle parts of your body to allow you to get the feeling back. You should move your feet, then your legs, and then your arms once the toes and fingers are finally coming back. You want to do this slowly, and take your time, because often it might take a little bit to get up.

9) You should then at this point go about the rest of your day. However, do have a set schedule to do this. You want to be consistent, which means not only the same length, but as well the same time. You

should have a set practice period in order to help you with getting the most out of your meditation. You should do it in small spurts than just one day a week for a long time, for the benefits will be much more apparent, and will come about much faster as well.

10) Finally, if you're not actually at home or in one space, you should start to figure out new places to meditate. There is no right or wrong place for you to meditate, but often it's based on your comfort level. Sure, meditating in the quietness of your home does a lot of good, but maybe you should try other locations, allowing you to become more aware of your surroundings, and it can even help you with your distractions. Some people love to meditate outdoors in nature, but you can also do it in your office chair, which is a great way to quell stress.

Figure out new places, and try it out, seeing what works for you.

These ten steps will allow you to have the best results from meditation, and it'll allow you to really get the most from this. If you've been worried about your meditation practices, do consider this method. It's a very simple way to get into the realm of meditation without too many stops or hurdles along the way.

For many, sitting down and trying to regulate breathing, mind, and their thoughts is a great means to improve oneself, but there is more out there for you to try. There are variants of these types of meditations, and they will be further explored in this chapter, including other techniques that you can use to help better yourself. By the end of this, you'll be able to understand and utilize various meditations that can help you out.

Open Monitoring Meditation

Instead of focusing, you will want to have your attention all out on the open, allowing you to monitor everything that is going on. You want to do all of this without judgment or any sort of attachment. Any perceptions that you might have, such as thoughts, feelings, memories, or external actions are seen for what they are.

This is the process of monitoring any content in the experience that you're sharing from every single movement. This is a variant of the meditation listed before, which wants you to focus, but if you are ready to look at meditation through a more open manner, this is the way to go.

Kindness Meditation

This is a form of meditation that encourages more kindness, goodwill, and benevolence. It does come from Buddhist traditions, and this form of compassion meditation does help with improving your ability to empathize with other people, making your emotions all the more positive and loving towards another, improving the acceptance of self, improving your competence about your life, and even giving more purpose to your own life.

Now to do it is simple. You simply sit down in the meditation position, with your eyes closed, and then, start to create feelings of kindness and benevolence. You should explore this within yourself, understanding what each of these are. Begin with yourself, generating this towards yourself, and from there, do it towards a close friend, a person that you're neutral about, someone that is difficult, doing this with all four of them with equal value, and then gradually move to the entire universe.

Now, this can be simply wishing that happiness and well-being is given to everyone. You can say various words to help create that boundless feeling of warm heartedness. You should visualize someone with problems and giving them love, or even imagining another person and wishing them happiness and good fortune.

For some, it's hard to find comparison and love for other people. Society has taught us to hate, to not show empathy, to not love even our enemies. However, the more that you do this, the better you'll be, and often, this can be seen as the secret to happiness. Try this, and see if it works for you.

Yoga Meditation

This is a type of meditation that is taught in yoga tradition, and this goes as far back as 1700 B.C, and it actually works to help improve your purification and your self-knowledge. Typically, classical yoga does divide this into various other facets, such as the rules, postures, and your breathing, along with some contemplation. You can try this, and often, the techniques can help you with improving your overall well-being.

How to do it is simple. The most common one is "third eye meditation" and this is essentially concentrating on a chakra point, mantra, visualization, or gazing meditation. It's a simple process, and anyone can do it.

- Third eye meditation is essentially focusing on that
  spot between where your eyebrows are. Once you
  have the attention constantly directed to that, it can
  actually silence the mind. By the time the gaps are
  actually focused on, they can get wider and deeper,
  increasing the presence as well. It is also
  accompanied by actually looking at this spot. For
  many, they tend to practice this for a few minutes,
  and it often yields some great results.
- Chakra: with chakra meditation, you're focusing on
  your chakras, which are the centers of energy. You
  can focus on the heart, your third eye, or even the
  crown chakras, which is at the top of the head. You
  can say various mantras as well, such as om, lam,
  ram, and vam. This can help you to put your focus on
  there. For many, they don't pay enough attention on
  these chakra points, and often, when they do realize

this, they can feel deeper feelings for a various point of themselves.

- Gazing: this is similar to the fixing attention meditation that is done, but it often can be done with the eyes open or closed, when typically with concentration meditation, the gaze is focused with the eyes open on the point. You want to typically use a cancel, and with the eyes closed, it can actually improve the visualization and the concentration of the mind. When you close your eyes, you can keep the image there in the place called the "mind's eye." You visualize this for a period of time. It's actually a very important form of meditation, and it can yield some great results.

- Kundalini: this is a much more complex practice. The goal of this is to get the kundalini energy, which is at the base of the spine, and this is actually what will start to awaken the various centers of the body, and enlistment. Now, this is a form of practice that you might want to try with a yogi, since it can be dangerous, and it's good to know about, but it definitely shouldn't be practiced willy-nilly

- Kriya yoga: this is a form of breathing, increasing your energy, and meditation that can help you with devotional temperament, and it can help with the spiritual aspects of meditation. This involves self-realization lessons that you can check out.

- Sound meditation: this is a very common yoga practice that you can try. You can focus on external sounds, and you will be able to collect your mind with this. To do this, you should start with meditation on an external sound. For this, you should choose some calming or ambient music and from there, you want to focus your attention hearing as a means to quiet and collect your mind. By the time you do this, you might end up hearing much deeper sounds, such as the body and the mind. Your goal is to hear a sound that is without vibration, which is manifested as "OM." This is one that you can do on your own, and while it might take a lot, it can definitely be worth learning.

Tantric Meditation

Now tantric in the western world has a much more sexual sort of intention behind it, with tantric massage being a sexual, but also very spiritual massage. However, there are actually meditations that you can employ to help create a stillness in your mind. However, with these, it's important that you master basic meditation first, since often, these are very hard to do, since it does require control. However, there are a few that you could try once you master basic meditation and focusing on yourself, and they are listed below:

- Take the mind and merge it with the senses into the interior of your spiritual heart
- When you perceive and object, notice that from this all objects become empty. Instead of concentrating on the object, concentrate on the emptiness
- Concentrate on that space between two specific thoughts
- Put your attention on the inside of the skull, and then close your eyes
- Meditation on the time of a great delight. Then, meditate on the feeling of pain
- Meditate and focus on the void of your body extending in all directions at the same time (for this one, it's encouraged that you have discovered the void before you attempt this)
- Concentrate on a bottomless well or standing at the edge of a very high place

- Concentrate intently on the idea of the universe being nothing

With this, you can even use Pranayama, which is breathing regulation. All other various forms of meditation can use this too, and you should try this before you begin any sort of meditation. Typically, it's in sequences of 4 sets of 4. In essence, you breathe in and count to four, hold this for about 4 seconds, and then breathe out for four seconds. Finally, you hold the empty void there for about 4 seconds. You should do this through the nose, all the way down to the abdomen, not just the chest cavity, and then out through your nose. You should have your abdomen move instead of the chest. With this, do it for a few cycles, and with this the breathing will balance out the mood and actually calm down the body. This alone can be done anywhere.

Self-Enquiry Meditation

This is the final, but also somewhat advanced form of meditation. Essentially, you're investigating the true nature of yourself, asking "who am I" and this can give you a very intimate knowledge of yourself in a way you've never thought possible. It does reference to older Indian texts, but it is a much modern form of meditation.

This is a very abstract practice, but it is also very subtle, and you'll be able to do it in a simple manner.

You see yourself at the center of the universe, also called the ego. It's the person behind all of your thoughts, mental pictures, and perceptions. In a sense, you're not totally clear on who the "I" is. You don't really know who you are in essence, and often, we confuse it with other labels, the roles we share, even our body and the memories that we have. If you think about it, it is a very deep mystery.

However, with self-enquiry meditation, you ask yourself "who am I?" at this point, you might get some verbal answers that might come, and you can reject these. You should focus on the feeling of fixing your attention on the subjective feeling of who you are. Start to become one with these feelings, getting in deep, truly looking at yourself. You will from this, learn who the true "I" is. This is a pure consciousness, beyond the limits, and it isn't an intellectual journey, but rather a way to bring to the forefront of who you are as a person. This isn't the personality, but it is the feeling of existing, without the concepts attached to it.

To do this, whenever you have thoughts or feelings arise, ask who brought these forward, and who is aware of these feelings. You will then realize it is yourself. From then you ask simply "who am I?" and then you get back to the feeling of self, of the presence that you have. In a sense, you're trying to get to the full level of awareness.

You can focus on the mind of the feeling of being, the yourself that shines within you. You should keep this pure, and don't associate it with anything in the outside world, or anything that isn't yourself.

This is a very deep and profound sense of meditation, since you are focusing deeply on yourself, and you might end up starting to realize more than you should have thought you could. You typically should have the meditation position for this, although there isn't a specific position for this. It's helpful for when you're starting on this type of deep meditation.

With meditation, there are many different methods out there, and you can further explore each of these yourself. While basic meditation was definitely focused on, and the branches of mindfulness and the like, understanding other types of meditation can help

broadening your horizons, and help you further

understand yourself and what your existence means as

well.

Conclusion

Meditation is a means to really help you explore your life, everything about it, and help with distractive thoughts. In a world where we take most things for granted, with an obsession over the material universe and positions, and even not paying much attention to our own bodies, in a sense, we need meditation. Meditation will allow us to indulge in a better and more conclusive understanding of the human spirit, and how our own spirituality can help us achieve greater happiness.

Meditation has been around for years for a good reason. It's a practice that can help a person in many different ways, allowing them to fully explore themselves and understand the various tidbits about yourself. We don't typically observe, but you'll notice that with meditation, it becomes almost natural for us to do, and it's something that you can use in order to fully understand, and for you to truly know what you're like.

With that being said, your next step is to try a few of these meditations. Begin with learning the basic meditations, and from there, start to go deeper. Work on understanding the nuances of your breathing, of how you regulate yourself, and of your mind. You'll begin to notice that this is actually a deep and profound process, and you'll begin to see that this is a new life for yourself. Try these, try to use them, and from there, you'll yield the full benefits of meditation that you so desire.